FROM CITRUS FRUIT
to
MEDICAL BREAKTHROUGH

The unique history and future of Modified Citrus Pectin

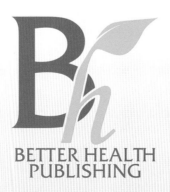

BETTER HEALTH
PUBLISHING

The purpose of this book is to educate. It is not intended to serve as a replacement for professional medical advice. Any use of the information in this book is at the reader's discretion. This book is sold with the understanding that neither the publisher nor the author has any liability or responsibility for any injury caused or alleged to be caused directly or indirectly by the information in this book. While every effort has been made to ensure its accuracy, the book's contents should not be construed as medical advice.

To obtain medical advice on your individual health needs, please consult a qualified health care practitioner.

Second Edition Copyright ©2014 Better Health Publishing

All rights reserved. No part of this publication may be reproduced, stored in a retrieval system, or transmitted in any form or any means, electronic, mechanical, photocopying, recording, or otherwise, without the prior written permission of the publisher.

Published by Better Health Publishing, Santa Rosa, CA

Printed in the United States of America

Contents

Foreword by Dr. Isaac Eliaz

"One day, they will find out that there is a cure for cancer in the peel of an orange."

I'll never forget these words. They came from Dr. Ruth Cohen, a neighbor of mine during my childhood in Israel 40 years ago. In a country known for its prized citrus fruits, she and her husband, Leo, were organic chemistry scientists with a particular focus on the study of citrus pectin.

Decades later, after becoming a doctor with a specialty in Integrative Cancer Treatments, I began to see how true Ruth's statement really was. What once seemed like mere wishful thinking had become a remarkable reality. In fact, a large body of scientific research now shows that a substance from the pith of citrus fruits, known as Modified Citrus Pectin (MCP), may well be one of the most important natural compounds to emerge in the last 20 years.

Today, there is a vast body of MCP research for cancer fighting properties *and* significant benefits for serious chronic conditions. My life's mission is to research and develop natural solutions that can fight disease and restore health, which is why I am excited about these discoveries that offer exciting new hope for everyone seeking safe and effective natural solutions.

In best health,

Isaac Eliaz, M.D., M.S., L.Ac.

Medical Director, Amitabha Medical Clinic

Modified Citrus Pectin

MCP Effectively Fights Cancer and More...

Many years of scientific and clinical research demonstrate that Modified Citrus Pectin (MCP) is a powerful and natural cancer fighter. Once known solely for this benefit, newer studies have established its value for inflammatory and fibrosis related conditions like cardiovascular disease, kidney disease, liver cirrhosis, diabetes and arthritis. This is because MCP is a natural blocker of Galectin-3.

In the last few decades, hundreds of studies have proven that Galectin-3 plays a role in cancer development. In small amounts, galectins are perfectly healthy and actually aid cellular communication, and healthy growth and development. However, studies show that excess Galectin-3 in the body directly promotes unhealthy cell behaviors such as inflammation, uncontrolled abnormal cell growth, colony formation (tumors) and metastasis, among others.

Because MCP is small enough to enter the bloodstream, and is naturally attracted to Galectin-3, it will bind and block over-expressed Galectin-3 molecules present in the body. This is the main mechanism by which MCP can prevent the growth and spread of cancer and other chronic degenerative conditions. In fact, Modified Citrus Pectin is the *only* natural substance proven to block excess Galectin-3 molecules in the body and prevent them from promoting cancer and other deadly diseases.

Other Unique MCP Benefits

In addition to addressing a number of specific health conditions, several clinical studies show that Modified Citrus Pectin can safely remove harmful heavy metals, radioactive isotopes and environmental toxins from the body. MCP's unique molecular structure makes it easily absorbed into the blood stream where it can safely and gently remove health robbing toxins without affecting essential mineral levels.

MCP has also been shown to activate the lymphocyte cells known as Natural Killer (NK) cells in human blood samples. NK cell activity has been demonstrated to destroy leukemia cells in culture.

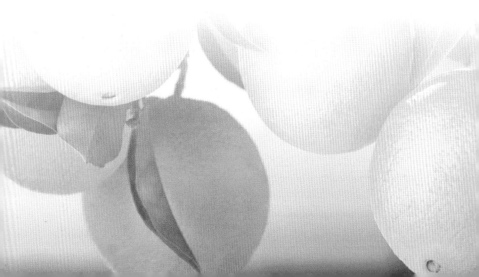

2

Science & Development

Regular Pectin versus Modified Citrus Pectin

We encounter unmodified pectin on a regular basis as a thickening agent for jams, jellies and other foods, yet the medical benefits of pectin are not widely recognized. On a basic chemistry level, pectin is a soluble fiber found in abundance in the peels of fruits like oranges, lemons, grapefruits and apples. Besides its usefulness in our diet, pectin actually provides a number of health benefits, especially in the digestive tract where it can help to remove toxins from the intestines and colon.

In the intestinal tract, pectin can bind and help remove mutagens which are harmful particles such as heavy metals, radioactive isotopes and environmental toxins capable of mutating DNA, disrupting cellular functions and wreaking havoc in the body. This is why pectin is known to reduce cancerous risks to your colon, and there are over a dozen published studies demonstrating this relationship.

While the benefits of pectin to the digestive tract have been understood for many years, its molecules are simply too large to provide benefits to other parts of the body. The additional disease-fighting properties in pectin remained untapped until the discovery of Modified Citrus Pectin.

Scientific Validation

In the ongoing search for a safe, natural substance useful in cancer therapy, Modified Citrus Pectin has emerged as one of the most promising. The first research on Modified Citrus Pectin was published in 1992 by Dr. Avraham Raz, a researcher at Wayne State University. Knowing the benefits of regular pectin, Dr. Raz was able to successfully demonstrate that a smaller pectin molecule could provide benefits in the fight against cancer.

Understanding the vital importance of these findings, a handful of doctors and researchers developed and standardized Modified Citrus Pectin — a natural pectin powder that is molecularly much smaller than regular pectin. With a smaller size, MCP's molecules can be easily absorbed into the bloodstream for maximum distribution throughout the body. Through this novel and safe modification, a flood of previously unknown health applications emerged, heralding a new chapter in the field of integrative cancer research.

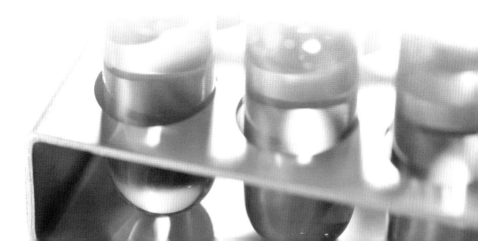

A Powerful Substance

Discussing the molecular composition of any substance can make for a complex topic. But since it is crucial to MCP's benefits, let's further explore the differences between regular pectin and Modified Citrus Pectin, and discuss the correct standards for an effective MCP.

Molecular Weight and Esterification

The size of pectin molecules ultimately determines where they can go and what they can do, and this value is expressed in terms of molecular weight, or *kilodaltons* (kDa). Regular pectin molecules are between 50 and 300 kilodaltons (kDa); far too large to enter the bloodstream and offer whole body health benefits.

To create an effective Modified Citrus Pectin, the proper method employs an enzymatic and pH process to yield an average molecular weight range between 3 and 15 kDa. This is the most scientifically proven and biologically active weight and the *only* MCP size that has been shown to be effective in human clinical trials.

Along with the correct molecular weight, another key factor to consider is the pectin's *degree of esterification* — and the rule of thumb is the smaller, the better.

Regular pectin has a degree of esterification of about 70 percent — but even some modified forms have as much as 50 percent, rendering it largely ineffective. The most powerful preparations of Modified Citrus Pectin have a degree of esterification of less than 10 percent. If the degree of esterification is too high, then the pectin chains link together and cross-bridge to each other, instead of blocking the harmful effects of Galectin-3.

When looking for the most effective MCP, the molecular weight needs to be between 3 and 15 kDa and the esterification should be below 10 percent.

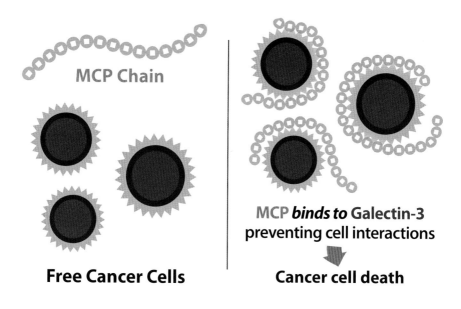

MCP Chain

Free Cancer Cells

MCP _binds to_ Galectin-3 preventing cell interactions

Cancer cell death

4

The Only Proven Natural Galectin-3 Inhibitor

How Galectin-3 Promotes Cancer

It's important to understand how cancerous cell behavior differs from normal, healthy cell behavior, so let's take a moment to explain some of the biological misfires involved in cancer's formation.

Healthy cells die and regenerate as part of an orderly cell cycle — as one dies, another is produced to replace it. When this cell cycle is disrupted, it causes cells to "pile up" and form a tumor. As long as these cells appear normal and static, the tumor is considered harmless or "benign."

Unlike benign tumors, cancerous tumors are malignant. They're marked by uncontrolled growth and the ability to spread aggressively, a process known as metastasis. Given the opportunity, they will spread through your entire body, invading healthy tissues and causing new tumors. And this dangerous ability hinges on the presence of excess Galectin-3.

Galectin-3 promotes cancer progression in 3 interconnected ways:

1. It allows cancer cells to attach to one another, forming groups that can survive in your bloodstream and migrate to other parts of your body.

2. Once cancer cells have formed a primary tumor, Galectin-3 allows the cells to aggregate and grow, and attach themselves to new sites as well, forming secondary tumors.

3. Galectin-3 nourishes malignant tumors by stimulating new blood vessel growth (even where there was no blood supply before) to feed the tumor. This process is called angiogenesis.

It's no surprise then that Galectin-3 molecules have become a therapeutic target in modern cancer prevention and treatment. If you disarm a cancer cell's ability to attach and communicate, you essentially pull the plug on its power supply. If it cannot spread or nourish itself, ultimately it will not proliferate or survive.

Modified Citrus Pectin's affinity to bind to Galectin-3 makes it a vital weapon in blocking the spread of cancer. By attaching to and blocking Galectin-3 on cancer cells' surface, MCP can disable their ability to communicate, nourish themselves and grow.

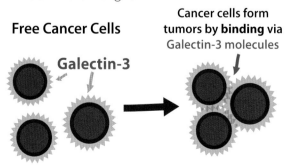

Free Cancer Cells

Galectin-3

Cancer cells form tumors by binding via Galectin-3 molecules

5

Prostate Cancer

Many men have benefited from the use of Modified Citrus Pectin before, during, and after a diagnosis of prostate cancer. As we'll discuss here, the body of MCP research for prostate cancer is quite impressive.

Dramatic Scientific Findings

In 1995, the first *in vivo* research studying the effects of MPC on prostate cancer metastasis was conducted by Dr. Kenneth J. Pienta. The results were excellent, showing a 56 percent decrease in lung metastasis — a significant difference. This important study was published in the prestigious *Journal of National Cancer Institute* (JNCI). Dr. Pienta's results paved the way for future MCP research, and the first human trial, a pilot study conducted by Dr. Isaac Eliaz along with Dr. Stephen Strum in 1995 and 1996, was presented at the International Conference on Diet and Prevention of Cancer in Finland in 1999.

In this pilot study, seven patients, with local recurrence of prostate cancer after local therapy, were administered 15 grams of MCP in three divided daily doses for 12 full months (15 grams daily is the standard recommended dose for cancer patients). During the study, PSA doubling time, a measurement that reflects the rate at which the cancer is growing, was evaluated at the three, six and twelve month mark and the results were extremely promising: four out of seven patients responded with a lengthened prostate specific antigen doubling time (PSADT) of more than 30 percent. Of the others, one patient was judged to have a partial response, one was judged to have stable disease and the remaining judged as having no response. Lengthening of the PSADT reflects a slowing down in the progression of the cancer.

Additional analysis using prostate cancer cells was also presented at the conference in Finland, revealing that MCP does indeed interfere with cancer cell growth and metastasis, resulting in cytotoxicity (cancer cell death) of 80.7 percent, compared with only 3.8 percent in the control.

Further Exploration and Results

Both of these studies warranted a longer and more controlled phase-II clinical study, which was completed in December 2003. This time, 10 patients with biochemical relapse of prostate cancer after local therapy were given 5 gram doses of MCP three times per day for a year. 70 percent of the participants showed positive response to this treatment, with a significant slowing in the rise of their PSA. In fact, six out of ten patients more than *doubled* their PSA doubling time — ultimately leading to a significant reduction in the chance of dying prematurely.

Columbia University Study

In 2010, research from Columbia University was published in the journal *Integrative Cancer Therapies* offering additional answers as to how Modified Citrus

Pectin achieves its remarkable anti-cancer effects. Laboratory results indicated that MCP can inhibit cell proliferation and promote apoptosis (programmed cell death) in prostate cancer cell lines (including androgen-dependent and androgen-independent cells). It was also shown to inhibit cell proliferation by reducing a cellular signaling process used by cancer to spread and proliferate throughout the body. This process is called mitogen-activated protein (MAP) kinase signaling.

The ability to induce apoptosis in androgen-independent prostate cancer cell lines is especially significant, as this is the more aggressive form of prostate cancer that can become resistant to treatment, metastasize and lead to premature death. Any help in slowing down the progression of this cancer obviously has a direct effect on prolonging a patient's life.

In closing, it must be said that even with all these significant benefits, Modified Citrus Pectin as a stand alone isn't a cure for prostate cancer.

But it *is* extremely valuable for any man in "watchful waiting" or "active surveillance" and a very important adjunct to standard treatment — not least of all because of the many unique benefits that continue to emerge with ongoing research into MCP use.

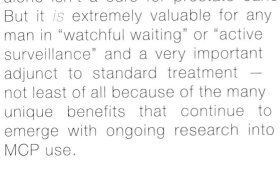

6

Breast Cancer & More

With breast cancer diagnoses at all time highs, the necessity of natural solutions is paramount. Fortunately, like its benefits for men with prostate cancer, Modified Citrus Pectin also has very important benefits for women.

In a 2002 in vivo breast cancer study, published in the *Journal of the National Cancer Institute*, Modified Citrus Pectin's effects on breast tumors were studied using varying doses. Results showed that MCP treatment inhibited tumor growth, angiogenesis and metastasis in mice (with larger doses yielding stronger results) via the blocking of Galectin-3. Earlier *in vitro* research supported these results revealing the same reduced angiogenesis (creation of new blood vessels that feed tumors) and cancer cell adhesion.

In addition to MCP's role in preventing and treating breast and prostate cancer, other MCP studies suggest that this versatile substance plays a crucial role in protecting against skin cancer. One study (published in the *Journal of the National Cancer Institute*) showed that while regular pectin demonstrated no positive effects on melanoma cells, the administration of MCP remarkably reduced tumor metastasis by over 90 percent. These incredible results were supported two years later in a follow-up study that demonstrated a similar decrease in melanoma progression. The study authors attributed this remarkable effect to MCP's superior Galectin-3 binding capabilities.

New Hope for Treatment Resistant Cancer

In 2008, a German study tracked a group of 49 patients with multiple types of cancer: colon, breast, lung cancer, pancreatic, ovarian, throat and others. These were not early-stage diagnoses. These patients had advanced cancers, most of which had metastasized. They had unsuccessfully gone through surgery, radiation therapy and chemotherapy.

And yet, 5 grams of Modified Citrus Pectin 3 times per day improved the quality of life and reduced pain in *the majority* (53 percent) of these patients. In fact, one patient with advanced prostate cancer had a *50 percent* decrease in his PSA level over the period of 16 weeks, with an equally significant decrease in his clinical symptoms and his pain. This is incredibly promising, especially for anyone who has been failed by available treatments.

Furthermore, the results of this study are equivalent to *and in some cases better than* the chemotherapy results achieved in the same group of patients — and without the toxicity and side effects. While MCP is not a replacement for conventional therapy, it is an integral part of a comprehensive program for cancer patients. It also quite possibly offers a new lease on life for anyone with advanced stage, treatment-resistant tumors.

Synergy: Combining Treatments

Integrative medicine demonstrates that the battle against cancer is best won by attacking it from multiple angles using synergistic anti-cancer therapies and treatments. Synergistic action means that different therapies work together and enhance each others beneficial effects. Here's a simple metaphor to explain synergistic action: with synergy, 1 + 1 equals not just 2, but 3, 5 or even 100, depending on which treatments are being used together. The strategic synergistic combination of various therapies is one of the keys to successful integrative health treatment.

Clinical observations and scientific studies show that MCP has the power to enhance chemotherapy and may also help the body to deal with some of chemotherapy's harmful side effects, which often further destroy a person's health. By using Modified Citrus Pectin in conjunction with traditional chemotherapy, a patient may receive the benefits of a synergistic action against the cancer. This synergy may allow for a lower dose of chemotherapy, less side effects and a greater clinical outcome. A synergistic anti-cancer effect has also been seen when MCP is used in conjunction with specialized botanical formulas to fight cancer and prevent metastasis via multiple mechanisms of action.

MCP is Critical Before and After Surgery/Biopsy

Cancer surgery or diagnostic biopsy is sometimes a necessary choice. If this is the case, MCP is a critical ally which can help protect against further damage potentially caused by these procedures. While cancer surgeries and biopsies may be necessary, they are not risk free. These procedures can create inflammation and damage to the surrounding tissue and circulation, increasing the potential for further growth and spread of the cancer. The injury to the tissue can increase inflammation and cause increases in various growth factors such as VEGF and EGF, both promoters of cancer growth. Surgery and biopsy can also increase the aggressive behavior of cancer cells, release them to migrate from the primary tumor site and invade other tissues, promoting metastasis.

That's where MCP can play a critical role in protecting against cancer proliferation, invasiveness and metastasis after surgery or biopsy. By taking 5 grams three times a day for two weeks prior, and two to four weeks after the procedure, patients can also reduce inflammation and abnormal scar tissue by relying on MCP's ability to bind and block Galectin-3. Some patients increase the dosage in the 24 hours before the procedure to 20-25 grams. Supplying an active dose of MCP before and after will help to protect against aggressive cancer cell behavior and potential metastasis following such a procedure.

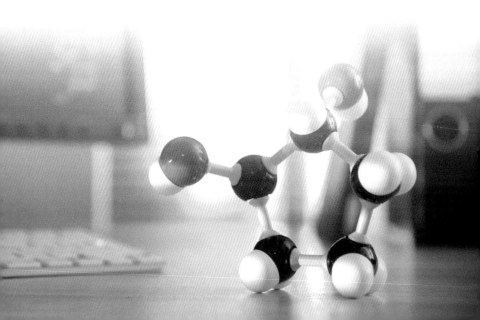

7

Heavy Metals & Radiation

Safely Chelate Toxic Metals and Radioactive Isotopes From Your Body for Improved Health

Another essential benefit of Modified Citrus Pectin is that it safely and gently chelates (tightly binds and removes) heavy metals and toxins from the body.

Heavy metals and toxins are a silent but serious health threat. Regrettably, we encounter toxins on a daily basis: there's mercury in amalgam dental fillings and in fish and seafood; lead in foods, old paint and water pipes; and numerous other heavy metals present in our air, water, soil and food chain. Even with the best efforts, it's nearly impossible to avoid some level of exposure, and even small amounts can accumulate in our body and contribute to the development of serious chronic illnesses.

Heavy metal toxicity can be seen in everything from chronic pain and high blood pressure to a variety of neuro-degenerative conditions and, most notably, cancer. Heavy metals distort cellular communication signals, mutate DNA, impair the immune system and disrupt numerous critical biological functions. Even if your heavy metal intake is limited to miniscule amounts at a time, these metals can build up gradually in bone and soft tissue, leading to very serious conditions down the road.

Given these harmful effects, the removal of toxic heavy metals is essential in reducing health risks, which is why the discovery of MCP's chelating powers presented such an exciting advancement in chelation and detoxification therapy. Once again, it's the unique molecular structure of MCP that provides the ability to remove these toxins, without removing essential minerals, as many other chelation agents unfortunately do.

MCP & the "Egg Box"

Modified Citrus Pectin belongs to a specific class of polysaccharides known as *polyuronides*. Studies on polyuronides demonstrate that they can remove heavy metals and toxins.

In solution, MCP's negatively-charged fiber chains stack together to create pockets, forming what we call an "egg box." Heavy metals have a strong positive charge and are attracted to these fiber chains, which cause the metal ions to bind to the pockets. Over time this process can stimulate a more thorough release of heavy metals and toxins from deep within your soft tissues where they're accumulating.

Once they come in contact with the "egg box," heavy metals become trapped and bound in the pockets, allowing them to be safely excreted from your body.

Mechanism of Action

Long fiber chains of Modified Citrus Pectin stack together, forming pockets where metal particles can become trapped in the fiber, like an "egg carton."

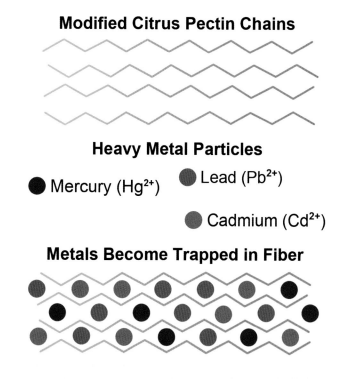

Modified Citrus Pectin Chains

Heavy Metal Particles

● Mercury (Hg^{2+})   ● Lead (Pb^{2+})

● Cadmium (Cd^{2+})

Metals Become Trapped in Fiber

Once the metals are bound to the fiber, they are removed from the body via the bloodstream or digestive system.

Pectin First Used in Chernobyl

Reports of pectin's remarkable effectiveness for toxin removal first surfaced during the efforts to minimize the devastating consequences of the Chernobyl disaster and radiation poisoning among local residents. In a multitude of cases, pectin prevailed as a powerful antidote to the toxic radiation by binding to the radioactive particles in the digestive tract and safely removing them. As the radiation fallout entered the food chains, children who received a diet which included pectin had significantly fewer cases of thyroid cancers than were occurring in the regions not receiving a pectin-rich diet.

Intrigued by the years of research following this natural approach to mitigating the effects of this overwhelming disaster, Dr. Isaac Eliaz headed a pilot study in collaboration with the United States Department of Agriculture (USDA) scientists to study Modified Citrus Pectin's ability to bind and remove toxic heavy metals. Not only were the results impressive, but they showed that MCP chelation does not disturb the body's essential mineral balance or cause any adverse side effects.

Clinical Studies on MCP and Heavy Metal Toxicity

Following the publication of this research with the USDA, Dr. Eliaz published a peer reviewed multiple case study report involving 5 patients from his clinic, Amitabha Medical Clinic and Healing Center in Sebastopol, California. Using MCP, it was the first study of its kind to show the relationship between heavy metal removal and the subsequent reduction of a wide range of clinical symptoms. In fact, not only did all five patients decrease their heavy metals by an impressive average of 74 percent, but participants' clinical symptoms ranging from elevating PSA levels to asthma, IBS, adrenal fatigue and depression, were significantly improved as heavy metal body burden was reduced over time. No adverse effects were reported. This affirming clinical evidence pointed to an important truth — namely, that heavy metals are a very prominent and deadly contributing factor in a wide range of serious health conditions.

In 2008, a study was published in the journal *Alternative Therapies in Health and Medicine*, demonstrating the effectiveness of using Modified Citrus Pectin as an antidote to acute lead poisoning in hospitalized children in China. These children all came from the same village where a battery producing plant was based. Their poisoning resulted in detectable levels of lead in their blood, and was enough to hospitalize them with symptoms.

The study followed their treatment with 5 grams of MCP 3 times a day for several weeks, and monitored their blood and urine lead content levels. They showed that their blood lead content levels decreased dramatically, and that lead was being expelled in their urine. All the children in the study saw a dramatic improvement and were able to be released from the hospital within three weeks, without side effects. Thankfully, the hospital involved in this study has reported that the battery plant in this village has since been shut down.

8

Heart Failure, Fibrosis, Immune Health & More

New Applications for MCP

As we discussed earlier, the understanding of MCP's value has grown significantly due to a number of key studies demonstrating the role of Galectin-3 in the progression of chronic diseases related to inflammation and fibrosis, including heart disease. Fibrosis is responsible for many chronic and deadly disease states because of the uncontrolled inflammation and subsequent overproduction of excessive scar tissue within various organs and systems.

Chronic Diseases

Arthritis

The finding that Galectin-3 is present in the inflamed joints of patients with rheumatoid arthritis strongly suggests that this protein is associated with the development and progression of this degenerative disease. Further research proves that Galectin-3 plays a large role in the development and progression of rheumatoid arthritis and that the disease severity is accompanied by harmful immune responses influenced by Galectin-3.

Diabetes

Diabetes resistance has also been linked to reduced Galectin-3. Mice with reduced Galectin-3 levels were shown through various measurements of diabetes progression to be resistant to the development of diabetes, as compared with mice that had normal levels of Galectin-3. The same mice with reduced Galectin-3 levels also showed a reduction in inflammation. Related research has demonstrated that reduction in Galectin-3 levels slows the breakdown of the inner blood-retinal barrier that typically occurs early in diabetes.

Liver Fibrosis

Inflammation and fibrosis of the liver has also been linked to excess Galectin-3.

Cardiac Diseases

Cardiovascular Disease

Using MCP to reduce Galectin-3 levels offers an important treatment option for cardiac diseases, particularly by reducing cardiac inflammation and fibrosis. Reducing Galectin-3 levels in the cardiac tissues of mice resulted in lowered inflammation and fibrosis in the cardiovascular system. Further studies suggest that lowering Galactin-3 levels following a heart insult or cardiac event can reduce or suppress cardiac fibrosis and heart disease.

FDA Approved Blood Test

Some of the most important recent research on Galectin-3 has demonstrated the link between high levels of Galectin-3 and chronic heart failure, giving value to

Galectin-3 as a biomarker of inflammation and fibrosis in patients with progressive heart disease. In 2010, the FDA approved a blood serum Galectin-3 test that is now available and covered by most medical insurances. This inexpensive tool helps to determine cardiovascular risks and disease prognosis, and can also be used to determine metastatic cancer risk and progression.

The Future of Galectin-3 Research

Due to new developments in Galectin-3 research, the relationship between Galectin-3 and many chronic health conditions is now highly documented. Galectin-3 research continues in other areas as well, such as gastrointestinal conditions, allergies and hypersensitivities, skin conditions, parasitic diseases, lung diseases (including asthma), and immune conditions including auto-immune diseases.

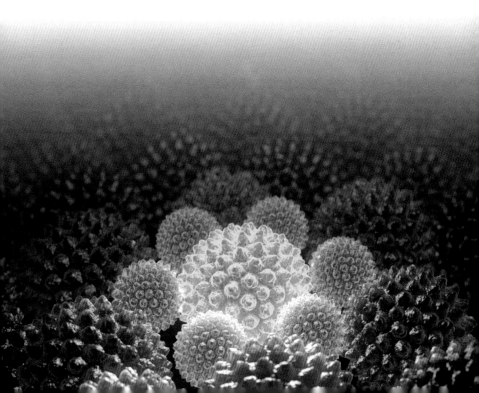

Galectin-3 Reference Ranges

This chart explains Galectin-3 test results which are measured as nanogram/milliliter (ng/ml).

Extreme Risk: >17.8	High Risk: 14.0 to 17.8	Ideal Levels: <14.0 to 12.0
Indicates high risk for cancer, heart failure and fibrosis in general populations. For congestive heart failure patients, these levels indicate extreme risk of adverse cardiac event.	Indicates significant increased risks for cancer, congestive heart failure, fibrosis and overall mortality.	General Population <14.0 ng/ml Cancer Patients <12.0 ng/ml Congestive Heart Falure Patients <12.0 ng/ml

- *Galectin-3 levels above 17.8 ng/ml are considered to be an extreme risk factor of mortality.*
- *Ideal levels are below 14 ng/ml in the general population.*
- *For cancer and cardiac patients, ideal levels are below 12 ng/ml.*
- *It's important to recognize that when levels change by 20% within 3 months, these changes correlate with increases or decreases in disease progression and mortality risk.*

For Galectin-3 testing information, please visit:
www.healthwisdomlabs.com

A Biomarker of Metastatic Cancer

Increased concentrations of free circulating Galectin-3 are commonly seen in the blood of many types of cancer patients including prostate, thyroid, gastric and colorectal cancer patients. Recent studies have shown that increases in circulating Galectin-3 levels in cancer patients contribute significantly to the metastatic spread of their cancer.

Increases in Galectin-3 levels enhance the cancer's ability to adhere to blood vessel walls and also avoid immune surveillance and detection. Results suggest that the interaction between free circulating Galectin-3 and cancer-associated *transmembrane mucin protein* (MUC1) promotes cancer cell clustering and the survival of tumor cells circulating in the body. By targeting and interrupting the interaction of circulating Galectin-3 with MUC1 proteins, Modified Citrus Pectin offers another effective mechanism of action for preventing cancer metastasis.

Powerful Immune Activation Properties

Another unique function of MCP was demonstrated in a 2011 study, showing its immune activation properties. Studies using human blood samples showed that MCP activated T-cytotoxic, B and Natural Killer (NK) immune cells in a leukemia model. NK cells play a major role in the rejection of tumors and cells infected by viruses. NK cells that were activated by MCP demonstrated increased functional ability in inducing cancer cell death among chronic myeloma leukemia cells. This research has paved the way for further investigation into these immune enhancement properties, and has also given science a more comprehensive understanding of MCP's potent cancer fighting properties. MCP supports appropriate immune response including powerful NK cell activation and increased functionality, essentially "tagging" the cancer cells for immune cell attack.

The Future of MCP

Ongoing validation of Modified Citrus Pectin's multiple health applications is helping integrative health care treatments world-wide. Thanks to the work of dedicated scientists, researchers and integrative doctors, the medical community and those interested in achieving and maintaining natural health will benefit from MCP in the treatment of a wide range of conditions. As research on this important substance continues, and as more health professionals and patients seek out effective natural solutions, Modified Citrus Pectin will surely be known as a very valuable substance involved in the maintenance of long term health and longevity.

As the only scientifically proven natural Galectin-3 blocker, Modified Citrus Pectin is important in the prevention and treatment of cancer, inflammation, cardiovascular disease and fibrosis, as well as being a valuable substance in the treatment of heavy metal toxicity, immune function and more. Thus, anyone concerned about the prevention, development and management of these conditions should consult their doctor about testing their levels of Galectin-3 and heavy metal body burden. Add daily MCP supplementation to your diet as an effective tool in preventing disease and maintaining long term health.

As promising new research on MCP's role in health and disease continues to emerge from the scientific community, future editions of this important body of knowledge will be updated to share with anyone seeking safe and effective natural health solutions.

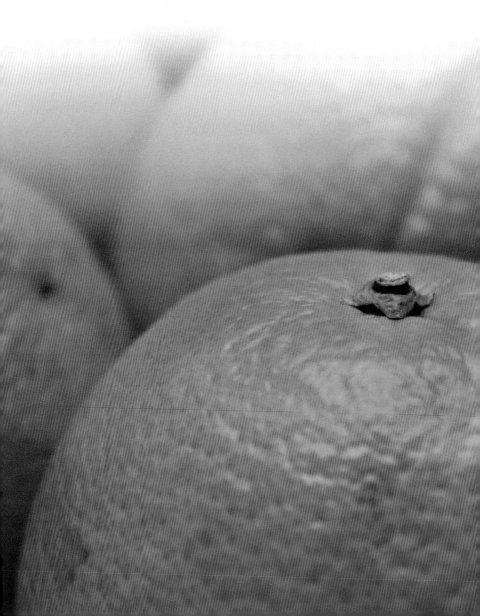

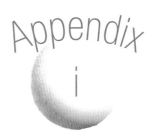

Appendix i

How to use MCP

MCP Dosage Per Day				
Galectin-3 Test Results	No Known Medical Conditions	Cardiovascular Inflammation Fibrosis Hepatitis	Active Cancer	Post-Cancer (3 Years)
<12 ng/ml	5 grams	5 grams	15 grams	5 grams
12-14 ng/ml	5 grams	10 grams	15 grams	10 grams
14-17.8 ng/ml	10 grams	15 grams	15 grams	15 grams
>17.8 ng/ml	15 grams	20 grams	20-25 grams	20-25 grams
Not Tested	5 grams	15 grams	15 grams	5-10 grams

MCP Dosage Per Day for Heavy Metal Toxicity				
Elevated levels of heavy metals (hair or urine analysis)	Frequent exposure to heavy metals	Low levels of heavy metals (hair or urine analysis)	Normal exposure to heavy metals, or for prevention	Cleansing and detoxification
15 grams	15grams	5 grams	5 grams	15 grams for 3-6 months

Frequently Asked Questions

What is the most effective way to dissolve Modified Citrus Pectin powder into liquid?

1. Put one 5 gram scoop of Modified Citrus Pectin into a glass.

2. Add your liquid (water, juice or tea).

3. Stir contents until powder is dissolved.

What is the best liquid to mix Modified Citrus Pectin powder with?

Water is best, but some people do use other liquids, such as juice. It's best to stir immediately upon adding the liquid and even better solubility results may be seen if using warm liquid. Modified Citrus Pectin has a very mild, bland taste.

What citrus fruits are used to make Modified Citrus Pectin?

The pectin contained in Modified Citrus Pectin is derived from lemons, limes, oranges and grapefruit. It is made from the pith of the fruit, no juice, pulp or any part of the "fruit" is used. Modified Citrus Pectin does not cause a "grapefruit" effect on absorption of medications.

What is the best way to store Modified Citrus Pectin?

Modified Citrus Pectin can be stored at room temperature; it is not necessary to store it in the refrigerator. Modified Citrus Pectin is a very stable material, and can withstand extreme temperatures.

Does Modified Citrus Pectin contain Vitamin C?

No, Modified Citrus Pectin does not contain any Vitamin C.

Is it okay to give Modified Citrus Pectin to my dog or cat?

Yes. Average, mid-sized dogs may take 1 scoop daily. Cats should take only ½ scoop, as they are smaller. It is usually best to mix it with your pets' fresh daily water.

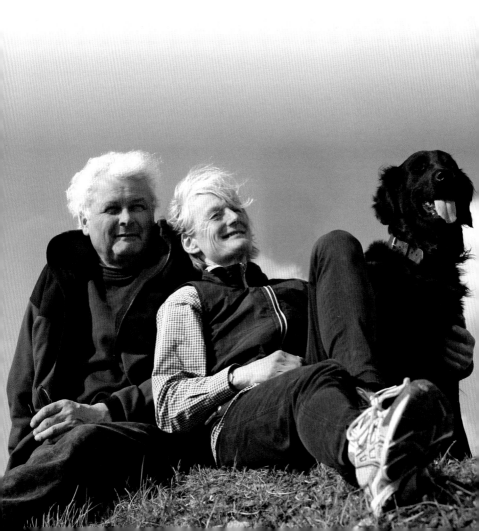

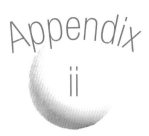

Appendix ii

References & Research

Abdou AG, Hammam MA, Farargy SE, Farag AG, El Shafey EN, Farouk S, Elnaidany NF. Diagnostic and prognostic role of galectin 3 expression in cutaneous melanoma. Am J Dermatopathol. 2010 Dec;32(8):809-14.

Azemar M, Hildenbrand B, Haering B, Manfred E. Heim, ME, Unger, C. Clinical benefit in patients with advanced solid tumors treated with modified citrus pectin: a prospective pilot study. Clinical Medicine: Oncology 2007:1 73-80.

Baekey PA, Cerda JJ, Burgin CW, Robbins FL, Rice RW, Baumgartner TG. Grapefruit pectin inhibits hypercholesterolemia and atherosclerosis in minature swine. Clin Cardiol, 1988:11(9):597-600.

Bereza Vla, Chaialo PP, Iatsula GS, Shimelis IV, Protas AF. Pectin-containing products in the dietary nutrition of subjects exposed to ionizing radiation as a result of the accident at the Chernobyl Atomic Electric Power Station. Lik Sprava, 1993 Jul; (8):21-4.

Breuilh L, Vanhoutte F, Fontaine J, van Stijn CM, Tillie-Leblond I, Capron M, Faveeuw C, Jouault T, van Die I, Gosset P, Trottein F. Galectin-3 modulates immune and inflammatory responses during helminthic infection: impact of Galectin-3 deficiency on the functions of dendritic cells. Infect Immun. 2007 Nov;75(11):5148-57.

Canning P, Glenn JV, Hsu DK, Liu FT, Gardiner TA, Stitt AW. Inhibition of advanced glycation and absence of Galectin-3 prevent blood-retinal barrier dysfunction during short-term diabetes. Exp Diabetes Res. 2007;2007:51837.

Cerda JJ, Normann SJ, Sullivan MP, Burgin CW, Robbins FL, Vathada S, Leelachaikul P. Inhibition of atherosclerosis by dietary pectin in microswine with sustained hypercholesterolemia. Circulation. 1994 Mar;89(3):1247-53.

Cerda JJ, Robbins FL, Burgin CW, Baumgartner TG, Rice RW. The effects of grapefruit pectin on patients at risk for coronary heart disease without altering diet or lifestyle. Clin Cardiol, 1988: 11:589-594.

Chen HY, Fermin A, Vardhana S, Weng IC, Lo KF, Chang EY, Maverakis E, Yang ,Y, Hsu DK, Dustin ML, Liu FT. Galectin-3 negatively regulates TCR-mediated CD4+ T-cell activation at the immunological synapse. Proc Natl Acad Sci U S A. 2009 Aug 25;106(34):14496-501.

de Boer RA, Voors AA, Muntendam P, van Gilst WH, van Veldhuisen DJ. Galectin-3: a novel mediator of heart failure development and progression Eur J Heart Fail. 2009;11:811-17.

de Boer RA, Yu L, van Veldhuisen DJ. Galectin-3 in cardiac remodeling and heart failure Curr Heart Fail Rep. 2010;7:1-8.

Eliaz I, Hotchkiss AT, Fishman ML, Rode D. The effect of modified citrus pectin on urinary excretion of toxic elements. Phytother Res. 2006 Oct;20(10):859-64.

Eliaz I, Gaurdino J, Hughes K: The health benefits of modified citrus pectin: in Patil BS, Brodbelt JS, Miller EG, and Turner ND (ed.): Potential health benefits of citrus. ACS Symposium Series 936. 2006: 199-210.

Eliaz I, Weil E, Wilk B. Integrative medicine and the role of modified citrus pectin/alginates in heavy metal chelation and detoxification—five case reports. Forsch Komplement Med. 2007 Dec;14(6):358-64.

Eliaz I. The potential role of modified citrus pectin in the prevention of cancer metastasis. Clin Practice Altern Med. 2001, Fall;2(3):177-179.

Forsman H, Islander U, Andréasson E, Andersson A, Onnheim K, Karlström A, Sävman K, Magnusson M, Brown KL, Karlsson A. Galectin 3 aggravates joint inflammation and destruction in antigen-induced arthritis. Arthritis Rheum. 2011 Feb;63(2):445-54.

Guess B, Scholz M, Strum S, Lam RY, Johnson HJ, Jennrich RI. Modified citrus pectin (MCP) increases the prostate specific antigen doubling time in men with prostate cancer: A Phase II clinical trial. Prostate Cancer Prostatic Dis. 2003;6(4):301-4.

Gunning, P, Bongaerts, RJM, Morris, VJ. Recognition of galactan components of pectin by Galectin-3. FASEB J. 2009, 23, 415–424.

Henderson NC, Mackinnon AC, Farnworth SL, Kipari T, Haslett C, Iredale JP, Liu FT, Hughes J, Sethi T. Galectin-3 expression and secretion links macrophages to the promotion of renal fibrosis. Am J Pathol. 2008 Feb;172(2):288-98.

Hexeberg S, Hexeberg E, Willumsen N, Berge RK. A study on lipid metabolism in the heart and liver of cholesterol- and pectin-fed rats. Br J Nutr, 1994, Feb, 71(2):181-92.

Honjo Y, Nangia-Makker P, Inohara H, Raz A. Down-regulation of Galectin-3 suppresses tumorigenicity of human breast carcinoma cells. Clin Cancer Res. 2001 Mar;7(3):661-8.

Hsu DK, Chen HY, Liu FT. Galectin-3 regulates T-cell functions. Immunol Rev. 2009 Jul;230(1):114-27.

Iacobini C, Menini S, Ricci C, Fantauzzi CB, Scipioni A, Salvi L, Cordone S, Delucchi F, Serino M, Federici M, Pricci F, Pugliese G. Galectin-3 ablation protects mice from diet-induced NASH: A major scavenging role for Galectin-3 in liver. J Hepatol. 2011 May;54(5):975-83.

Inohara H, Raz A. Effects of natural complex carbohydrate (citrus pectin) on murine melanoma cell properties related to Galectin-3 functions. Glycoconj J, 1994; 11(6): 527-32.

Jiang, J, Isaac Eliaz, I, Sliva, D. Synergistic effect of modified citrus pectin with two novel poly botanical compounds, in the suppression of invasive behavior of human breast and prostate cancer cells. 2011 (Submitted for Publication).

Johnson KD, Glinskii OV, Mossine VV, Turk JR, Mawhinney TP, Anthony DC, Henry CJ, Huxley VH, Glinsky GV, Pienta KJ, Raz A, Glinsky VV. Galectin-3 as a potential therapeutic target in tumors arising from malignant endothelia. Neoplasia. 2007 Aug;9(8):662-70.

Kolatsi-Joannou, M, Price, KL, Winyard, PJ, Long, DA. Modified citrus pectin reduces Galectin-3 expression and disease severity in experimental acute kidney injury. PLoS ONE 6(4): e18683. doi:10.1371/journal.pone.0018683

Li W, Jian-jun W, Xue-Feng Z, Feng Z. CD133(+) human pulmonary adenocarcinoma cells induce apoptosis of CD8(+) T cells by highly expressed Galectin-3. Clin Invest Med. 2010 Feb 1;33(1):E44-53.

Lin YH, Lin LY, Wu YW, Chien KL, Lee CM, Hsu RB, Chao CL, Wang SS, Hsein YC, Liao LC, Ho YL, Chen MF. The relationship between serum Galectin-3 and serum markers of cardiac extracellular matrix turnover in heart failure patients. Clin Chim Acta. 2009 Nov;409(1-2):96-9.

Mensah-Brown EP, Al Rabesi Z, Shahin A, Al Shamsi M, Arsenijevic N, Hsu DK, Liu FT, Lukic ML. Targeted disruption of the Galectin-3 gene results in decreased susceptibility to multiple low dose streptozotocin-induced diabetes in mice. Clin Immunol. 2009 Jan;130(1):83-8.

Miyazaki J, Hokari R, Kato S, Tsuzuki Y, Kawaguchi A, Nagao S, Itoh K, Miura S. Increased expression of Galectin-3 in primary gastric cancer and the metastatic lymph nodes. Oncol Rep. 2002 Nov-Dec;9(6):1307-12.

Müller S, Schaffer T, Flogerzi B, Fleetwood A, Weimann R, Schoepfer AM, Seibold F. Galectin-3 modulates T cell activity and is reduced in the inflamed intestinal epithelium in IBD. Inflamm Bowel Dis. 2006 Jul;12(7):588-97.

Nangia-Makker P, Hogan V, Honjo Y, Baccarini S, Tait L, Bresalier R, Raz A. Inhibition of human cancer cell growth and matastasis in nude mice by oral intake of modified citrus pectin. J Natl Cancer Inst, 2002; 94:1854-62.

Nangia-Makker P, Honjo Y, Sarvis R, Akahani S, Hogan V, Pienta KJ, Raz A. Galectin-3 induces endothelial cell morphogenesis and angiogenesis. Am J Pathol. 2000 Mar;156(3):899-909.

Oakley MS, Majam V, Mahajan B, Gerald N, Anantharaman V, Ward JM, Faucette LJ, McCutchan TF, Zheng H, Terabe M, Berzofsky JA, Aravind L, Kumar S. Pathogenic roles of CD14, Galectin-3, and OX40 during experimental cerebral malaria in mice. PLoS One. 2009 Aug 27;4(8):e6793.

Pienta KJ, Naik H, Akhtar A, Yamazaki K, Replogle TS, Lehr J, Donat TL, Tait L, Hogan V, Raz A. Inhibition of spontaneous matastasis in a rat prostate cancer model by oral administration of modified citrus pectin. J Natl Cancer Inst, March 1, 1995, 1:87(5):348-53.

Platt D, Raz A. Modulation of the lung colonization of B16-F1 melanoma cells by citrus pectin. J Natl Cancer Inst, 1994; 84(6):438-42.

Psarras S, Mavroidis M, Sanoudou D, Davos CH, Xanthou G, Varela AE, Panoutsakopoulou V, Capetanaki Y. Regulation of adverse remodeling by osteopontin in a genetic heart failure model. Eur Heart J. 2011 Apr 26. [Epub ahead of print]

Ramachandran, C, Wilk, BJ, Hotchkiss, A, Chau, H, Eliaz, I. Melnick, SJ. Activation of human T-helper/inducer cell, T-cytotoxic/suppressor cell, B-cell, and natural killer (NK)-cells and induction of natural killer cell activity against K562 chronic myeloid leukemia cells with modified citrus pectin. 2011. (Submitted for Publication).

Romanenko AE, Dereviago IB, Litenko VA, Obodovich AN. Further improvement in the administration of pectin as a preventive agent against absorption of radionuclides by human body. Gig Tr Prof Zabol, 1991;(12):8-10.

Saegusa J, Hsu DK, Chen HY, Yu L, Fermin A, Fung MA, Liu FT. Galectin-3 is critical for the development of the allergic inflammatory response in a mouse model of atopic dermatitis. Am J Pathol. 2009 Mar;174(3):922-31.

Sethi K, Sarkar S, Das S, Mohanty B, Mandal M. Biomarkers for the diagnosis of thyroid cancer. J Exp Ther Oncol. 2010;8(4):341-52.

Sioud M, Mobergslien A, Boudabous A, Fløisand Y. Evidence for the involvement of Galectin-3 in mesenchymal stem cell suppression of allogeneic T-cell proliferation. Scand J Immunol. 2010 Apr;71(4):267-74.

Strum,S, Scholz, M, McDermed, J, McCulloch, M, Eliaz, I. Modified citrus pectin slows PSA doubling time: A Pilot Clinical Trial. International Conference on Diet and Prevention of Cancer. 1999 Tampere, Finland.

Vagnucci Jr AH, Li WW. Alzheimer's disease and angiogenesis. The Lancet. Feb 15, 2003.

Vankrunkelsven A, De Ceulaer K, Hsu D, Liu FT, De Baetselier P, Stijlemans B. Lack of Galectin-3 alleviates trypanosomiasis-associated anemia of inflammation. Immunobiology. 2010 Sep-Oct;215(9-10):833-41.

Weiss, T, McCulloch, M, Eliaz, I. Modified citrus pectin induces cytotoxicity of prostate cacner cells in co-cultures with human endothelial monolayers. International Conference on Diet and Prevention of Cancer. 1999 Tampere, Finland.

Wang CR, Shiau AL, Chen SY, Cheng ZS, Li YT, Lee CH, Yo YT, Lo CW, Lin YS, Juan HY, Chen YL, Wu CL. Intra-articular lentivirus-mediated delivery of Galectin-3 shRNA and galectin-1 gene ameliorates collagen-induced arthritis. Gene Ther. 2010 Oct;17(10):1225-33.

Wang, Y, Nangia-Makker, P, Larry Tait, T, Vitaly Balan, V, Victor Hogan,V, Kenneth J. Pienta, KJ, Raz, A. Regulation of prostate cancer progression by Galectin-3. Am J Pathol. 2009 Apr;174(4):1515-23.

Yan, J, and Katz, AE. PectaSol-C modified citrus pectin induces apoptosis and inhibition of proliferation in human and mouse androgen-dependent and- independent prostate cancer cells. Integr Cancer Ther 2010;9:197-203.

Yu, LJ. Circulating Galectin-3 in the bloodstream: An emerging promoter of cancer metastasis. World J Gastrointest Oncol. 2010 ; 2(4):177-180.

Zhao, Z. Y., Liang, L., Fan, X., Yu, Z., Hotchkiss, A.T., Wilk, B. J., Eliaz, I. The role of modified citrus pectin as an effective chelator of lead in children hospitalized with toxic lead levels. Altern Ther Health Med. 2008;(4):34-38.

Zhao, Q, Barclay, M, Hilkens, J, Xiuli Guo, X , Barrow, H, Rhodes, JM, Yu, LG. Interaction between circulating Galectin-3 and cancer-associated MUC1 enhances tumour cell homotypic aggregation and prevents anoikis. Molecular Cancer. 2010, 9:154-166.

Zuberi RI, Hsu DK, Kalayci O, Chen HY, Sheldon HK, Yu L, Apgar JR, Kawakami T, Lilly CM, Liu FT. Critical role for Galectin-3 in airway inflammation and bronchial hyperresponsiveness in a murine model of asthma. Am J Pathol. 2004 Dec;165(6):2045-53.

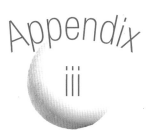

Appendix iii

Index